Ana Beatriz Teodoro Borges
Anna Luiza Pires Vieira
Lara Santos Brusamolin

Welcoming siblings of patients admitted to a neonatal ICU

Ana Beatriz Teodoro Borges
Anna Luiza Pires Vieira
Lara Santos Brusamolin

Welcoming siblings of patients admitted to a neonatal ICU

Humanization Project

ScienciaScripts

Imprint

Any brand names and product names mentioned in this book are subject to trademark, brand or patent protection and are trademarks or registered trademarks of their respective holders. The use of brand names, product names, common names, trade names, product descriptions etc. even without a particular marking in this work is in no way to be construed to mean that such names may be regarded as unrestricted in respect of trademark and brand protection legislation and could thus be used by anyone.

Cover image: www.ingimage.com

This book is a translation from the original published under ISBN 978-613-9-62779-0.

Publisher:
Sciencia Scripts
is a trademark of
Dodo Books Indian Ocean Ltd. and OmniScriptum S.R.L publishing group

120 High Road, East Finchley, London, N2 9ED, United Kingdom
Str. Armeneasca 28/1, office 1, Chisinau MD-2012, Republic of Moldova, Europe
Printed at: see last page
ISBN: 978-620-7-75087-0

index:

Humanization Project: Welcoming the siblings of patients admitted to a neonatal intensive care unit at a teaching hospital

Humanization Project: Reception of siblings of patients hospitalized in a hospital-school neonatal intensive care unit Aluizio Alvarenga, Ana Beatriz Teodoro Borges, Anna Luiz Pires Vieira, Bruna Teles da Silva, Cilene Fagundes, Edgar Loureiro Laborne de Mendonça, Jussara Paula de Oliveira, Lara Santos Brusamolin, Raissa Ritielle Olivia Cruz

1- Summary:

The Program to Welcome the Siblings of Babies Admitted to the Neonatal Intensive Care Unit (NICU) of a Public Hospital emerged in 2016, based on the demand presented by the mothers, who observed a lot of anguish and psychic suffering due to the change in behavior presented by their healthy children who remained at home, such as insecurities, fears, irritability and insomnia. This program was created in order to strengthen the maternal and family bond and promote humanization and welcoming. The aim of this study was to report on the experience of the method of welcoming the siblings of patients admitted to the neonatal unit of a teaching hospital. The methodology was a descriptive observational study, with the observation and reporting of the mothers of patients admitted to the NICU. Sibling visits were stipulated for children aged between 3 and 11, an age that is not routinely allowed in the NICU. Visits take place weekly, at set times, under the supervision and guidance of the neonatology and psychology departments. Before the visits, the parents and siblings go through an assessment with the psychologist, regarding their expectations and anxieties about the hospitalized child. During the visits, the children stay as long as they want, and are encouraged to talk, ask questions and do play activities with their siblings, such as singing and drawing pictures. After the visit, the psychology team approaches the children and their parents again, asking about their doubts and their satisfaction with the experience. In the one year since the program was set up, 40 children have been taken in. None of the children reacted strangely or negatively to the experience. They all asked to return to visit their siblings. During the course of the hospitalization, the parents reported to the psychologist about behavioral changes in their healthy children, such as sleep, aggression, eating habits and anxiety about discharge and the illness of their hospitalized sibling. The experience of visiting small siblings in the NICU made it possible to ease the mother's anxieties and anxieties about her small child at home, dispelling feelings of guilt and abandonment of her healthy children. In addition, the young child feels like an active participant in their sibling's hospitalization process.

Keywords: Reception, family, neonatal intensive care.

2- Introduction:

Preterm birth is a relatively common phenomenon in Brazil, accounting for 11.7% of births in 2010, according to research led by the Federal University of Pelotas (UFPel) in partnership with twelve other universities in the country, the United Nations Children's Fund (UNICEF) and the Ministry of Health. Premature babies are very vulnerable, as they are not yet ready for life outside the womb and most of the time need to stay in hospital in the Neonatal Intensive Care Unit (NICU). It is therefore important to emphasize that prematurity is the main cause of NICU admissions, but any newborn may need this environment as a result of some complication.

Hospitalization in the NICU has an impact on the newborn, as they are introduced to an inhospitable environment, with intense and frequent exposure to stimuli such as stress and pain. It represents the maximum expression of vulnerability, requiring organic and psychological rescue and, therefore, a great deal of support, especially from the family.

However, the family also suffers the consequences of this situation. Normally, the arrival of a child is synonymous with transformations within the family, whether it's a change in roles and responsibilities, or the anguish and fear that something might go wrong. This is aggravated by the fact that a newborn's stay in a NICU is often associated with seriousness and the possibility of death.

Another difficulty that many families face when a newborn is admitted to an intensive care unit is how the older siblings cope. Many of them don't understand why their newborn is in hospital for so long and wonder why their younger sibling has to stay there for so long, when they will return home or if they will even be able to play.

This extended stay in hospital can also cause older siblings to suffer from sleeping and eating disorders, difficulties at school, in their daily routine and in their social relationships. It can also lead to bouts of jealousy, which can be revealed by aggressive behavior or even excessive attachment. They may also be curious and anxious about the baby.

It is believed that these feelings are mainly due to the mother's greater absence, since even when she is with her older son, her feelings and worries are concentrated on the hospitalized baby, which is transmitted in some way to her brother. This means that even when the mother is physically present, she may not be emotionally available.

Against this backdrop, the importance of family visits in the NICU has become increasingly evident, mainly due to the greater value given to humanization, encompassing not only parents, but also siblings and grandparents, for example.

This practice has been endorsed mainly by the Standard of Humanized Care for Low Weight Neonates, which translates into the *Kangaroo Method*, launched by the Ministry of Health. This standard makes it easier for parents and other family members, such as siblings, to enter the neonatal ICU. In the United States, it is also recommended by the American Academy of Pediatrics.

In Brazil, the first program that advocated visits from siblings in the NICU was "Lembam-se de mim!" (They remembered me!), implemented in 1996 in a Neonatal Intensive Care Unit of a private clinic in Rio de Janeiro. Based on this model and on the recommendations of the Ministry of Health through the Kangaroo Method, a project was started in April 2016 to welcome siblings, aged 3 to 11, of newborns admitted to the Neonatal Intensive Care Unit of the Samuel Libânio Clinical Hospital in the city of Pouso Alegre. This experience was analyzed over a period of one year.

Visits by the sib ings of hospitalized newborns take place under the supervision of the hospital's neonatology and psychology department. Before the visits, the parents and siblings undergo an assessment with the psychologist, regarding their expectations and anxieties about the hospitalized child. During the visit, the children are encouraged to talk and interact with their siblings, doing activities such as singing and drawing pictures, and they can stay as long as they like. After the visit is over, the psychology department evaluates the child's impressions, doubts and satisfaction with the experience.

3- Objective:

The aim of this article is to describe the experience of the method of welcoming the siblings of patients admitted to the neonatal unit of a teaching hospital.

4- Methods:

The setting for the study was the Neonatal Intensive Care Unit (NICU) of the Samuel Libânio Clinical Hospital in Pouso Alegre, Minas Gerais. The study period was one year (April 2016 to April 2017). This was a descriptive observational study, using the methodology of observing and reporting on the mothers of patients admitted to the NICU. The observational criteria included monitoring behavior, play, drawings, the use of toys, reactions and gestures, as well as their meanings. Thus, in order to understand the fraternal relationship in a situation of family crisis due to the illness or fragility of one of its members, all of the siblings' expressions were valued. The bases of developmental psychology were used, with paradigms of the evolutionary range, and clinical psychology in the understanding of crisis situations, hospitalization, rivalry, signs of aggression, depression, among others. All the information was collected in the care area of the institution by the psychologist in charge, who act vely participated in the meetings with the siblings and kept records in a field diary.

Sibling visits were stipulated for children aged between 3 and 11, an age that is not routinely allowed in the NICU. Visits take place weekly, at set times, under the supervision and guidance of the hospital's neonatology and psychology departments. Before the visits, the parents and siblings undergo an assessment with the psychologist, regarding their expectations and anxieties about the hospitalized child. The psychologist may suggest play activities and drawings so that, feeling protected by the play activities, they can talk about their feelings and perceptions. Before entering the NICU, the children are instructed on antisepsis, especially of the hands, and are properly dressed. During the visits, the children stay as long as they want and are encouraged to talk, ask questions and do play activities with their siblings, such as singing and drawing pictures (they can give the babies the drawings they made at the first moment). After the visit, the psychology team approaches the child and parents again, asking about their doubts and their satisfaction with the experience. The psychology team tries to facilitate the visiting child's communication with the team, explain how the equipment used by the baby works, answer their questions, assess the need for other interventions and allow the family to find their own ways of experiencing this encounter. During their sibling's stay in hospital, the family, especially the mother, is accompanied by the psychologist, who reports on her own and her siblings' reactions to the late-night visit.

5- Results:

In the one year since the program was set up, 40 children have been taken in. Based on the methods used in this study, we found that no child reacted strangely or negatively to the experience. No stress behaviors were observed in the children who took part in the program's activities, either during or after the visit. On the contrary, it was noticed that when they felt welcomed and guided, they received support to cope with the situation.

At the beginning of the project, when they were introduced to the program, parents questioned the appropriateness and objectives of bringing their older siblings to visit. The doubt stemmed from the child's young age and their ability to understand what was happening with their hospitalized sibling. When faced with the baby and the devices, such as the probes, the respirator, the catheter or the monitoring itself, the children could project worry or fright, thus raising possible harm for these siblings. In view of this, the team responsible for the project offered all the necessary guidance so that the parents could decide whether or not to participate in the program and when they wanted to, and even if they did, the children would only come for the visit if they so decided, after the psychologist's initial approach.

The age range of the older sibling and its relationship to behavior during the visit is notable in this study. Smaller children usually arrive anxiously at the incubator and feel the need to touch the baby, questioning its movements and expressions. Older children are more observant, ask questions about the NICU routine or the patient's progress, such as when they will be discharged and if they are getting better, usually stay until the end of the visit, use more artifacts in their interaction with their sibling and get more emotional.

After the visits began, the reports collected by the psychology department revealed how much the siblings' visit allowed the family to come together in the neonatal intensive care environment, and to recover the roles of each of its members. It was noticed that the families whose children actively participated in the program remained in more frequent contact after discharge, sending news and reports affirming the importance of this work. These children proved to be more active in the post-discharge care process, as we observed, for example, in newborns with syndromes or malformations, for whom the visits helped their siblings prepare for the new demands of this family history. None of the children we visited died in our work, so the experience and reaction of the siblings in this specific situation is not reported.

In the reality of the older siblings, when the lack of information about the hospitalization forms fantasies about their guilt in the occurrence of the baby's risk situation, no stress behaviors were observed in the children who took part in the program's activities. The initial assessment, which included playwork, proved to be a space for doubts and feelings to be expressed, according to the different age groups, and previously worked on.

During the course of the hospitalization, the parents told the psychologist about behavioral changes in their healthy children, such as a reduction in complaints at school and the disappearance of psychosomatic disorders that arose after the baby was born. Parents often report that, after the visits, their older children encourage the mother and father to stay in hospital. In addition, it was observed that the visit of the eldest child allowed the parents to reduce the idea of the newborn's great fragility, which made it easier for the parents to be close to them. All the children asked to come back again to visit their hospitalized siblings.

The hospitalized newborns, all of whom were stable at the time of the visit, reacted as expected during the visits, with the medical team reporting a more favorable evolution as a result of this greater establishment of the family bond. After discharge, the child's reception and care at home was made easier by the reaction and care of the siblings who took part in the project. The health team reported that the visits did not interfere negatively with the clinical care (medical and nursing) provided to the child, but on the contrary made humanization more real in the NICU environment. With the program, the team is able to give the patient an identity, getting to know their family better. Because of the way the project is run, with all the support from the team, the patient reported that the visits minimized all the risks of stress that could arise in the siblings with the scope of risk that the family is being exposed to. According to the reports collected from health professionals, welcoming the family, in the ICU or any other neonatal or pediatric hospitalization unit, is not just about allowing the parents or a relative, such as the sibling, to enter and stay in the unit, but about establishing a relationship of trust and sincerity between the team, the family and the child; providing the means for parents and siblings to be included in the child's care process, taking on the role of educators, clarifying doubts and preparing the parents' family for the hospital discharge process.

The project detailed here represents the visits made to patients in the Neonatal ICU at the teaching hospital. The mothers gave their permission for photographs to be taken of some of the visits in order to show the work better. Annex II contains some images, also authorized, of the view of the siblings of patients admitted to the Pediatric ICU of the same teaching hospital, a project that was in line with the one reported in this study.

6- Discussion:

Due to technical and scientific advances in the health field, care has become increasingly disease-centered, detached from the person who houses it and in whom it develops. As a result, patients are often seen as objects of technical intervention, and their anxieties, expectations and fears are disregarded in the treatment process, causing human dignity to be relegated to second place.

In view of the damage that this scenario can cause, the attempt to humanize hospitals has been gaining ground. For humanization to be effective, it is necessary to reflect on the principles and values that coordinate professional practice so that dignified, welcoming and supportive patient care is guaranteed. It is a slow and complex process, as it involves adapting to changes in behavior.

According to the National Program for the Humanization of Hospital Care (PNHAH), regulated by the Ministry of Health, humanization can only happen through a collective effort by multi-professional teams, aimed at identifying the needs and interests of those involved. In the hospital environment, it must be based on the principle that the patient needs to continue to be seen as a human being, in other words, their anxieties and anxieties need to be respected, regardless of the reason why they are in hospital.

It has already been observed and reported that by improving the hospital environment through humanization, there are benefits such as reduced length of stay, increased general well-being of patients and healthcare staff and reduced staff absenteeism which consequently leads to lower costs for the hospital.

In view of all these benefits, humanization projects began to emerge a few years ago. Thus, allied to the knowledge of the high number of low birth weight neonates (weighing less than 2500g) and the high percentage of neonatal morbidity and mortality, the Kangaroo Method was created, which integrates Humanized Care for the Low Birth Weight Newborn.

The aim of this project is to improve the quality of care provided to newborns, their families and pregnant women. The aim is to guarantee a shorter hospital stay for the baby, increase the family's bond with the hospital staff, reduce the time the baby and family are apart, control and relieve pain and stress, stimulate the baby's development, reduce crying, increase body temperature and stability, improve the quality of the newborn's neurobehavioral and psycho-affective development, reduce the number of readmissions and enable parents to be more competent and confident in caring for their child after discharge.

The presence of the mother accompanying the hospitalized newborn is a source of protection, support and security for the child and enables closer emotional bonds, stress reduction, contributing to a better recovery and shorter hospital stay. However, family dynamics are affected when faced with the binomial illness of the child - absence of the mother. Expectations of the newborn's arrival change to insecurity about being hospitalized. And it is difficult for older siblings to understand this context without anguish and anxiety. With a view to alleviating this reality, our project was designed, based and initiated, reaping surprising results through this intervention.

The Program to Welcome the Siblings of Babies Admitted to the Neonatal Intensive Care Unit: "Remember Me!", implemented in a Neonatal Intensive Care Unit of a private clinic in Rio de Janeiro in 1996, represents one of the activities encouraged by the Kangaroo Method. This program was a pioneer in Brazil in terms of its model, although similar programs already existed elsewhere in the world, such as in the United States of America, and were recommended by the American Academy of Pediatrics.

The initiative for this program came about at the request of the babies' siblings, who were curious to meet them and worried about seeing their parents more distant and distressed due to their newborn's hospitalization. As a result, the parents also complained that the older siblings were beginning to have eating disorders, sleep problems, difficulties at school and in carrying out their usual activities, as well as appearing anxious and afraid.

In this way, "They remembered me!" aims to involve the siblings in the baby's hospitalization process, informing them about the patient's clinical condition and needs, so that there is a better understanding and offering greater support for the older sibling to continue carrying out their daily activities normally and not be affected by aggressive feelings, sadness and guilt over the situation the baby is in.

This program does not restrict the age of the siblings who will make the visits and does not segregate those with cognitive deficits, psychological problems or even more serious developmental disorders. Weekly visits last two hours and are divided into three parts.

First of all, the sibling is welcomed, their doubts are clarified and they are encouraged to prepare drawings and activities for the hospitalized baby, so that they can express their feelings and perceptions.

Secondly, the children are instructed on asepsis and are taken to their brother with what they made at the first moment. They spend around twenty minutes in the Intensive Care Unit and, during the process, the psychology team tries to make the moment as peaceful as possible, explaining how the equipment works, answering questions and thus facilitating the visitor's communication with their brother.

Finally, the older siblings talk about their experience with the psychology team, showing the positive and negative aspects of the process.

It was observed that, with these visits, having the family together in a Neonatal Intensive Care Unit makes it possible to rescue and determine the function of each of its members. In addition, parents lose some of the idea of their baby's fragility, reducing their fear of touching or talking to them. The post-discharge period for these hospitalized newborns was also more interesting, as the parents began to send more news, reinforcing the importance of the project. And in families where the newborns have malformations or syndromes, the visit prepares the siblings for the new reality that the family will have to face.

The siblings showed no stress behaviors during the project. After the visits, the parents reported that the bad feelings and behaviors caused by their newborn's hospitalization had disappeared, and their performance at school had improved. Drawing pictures and carrying out play activities before the visits proved to be a providential factor for the older siblings to express their doubts and feelings and help the psychologists to better manage the situation.

From observing these facts, it can be seen that the initiative to take in older siblings is decisive for the start of the fraternal bond and for the parents' greater peace of mind during the newborn's hospitalization. The little patient is seen as less fragile by the family members and the feelings of guilt, sadness, anguish and denial of the situation are replaced by hope and give them more strength to believe in the importance of continuing treatment.

One of the activities encouraged and carried out during the visits was music, when the older siblings sang to the younger ones, making them feel more comfortable. As reviewed in the literature, in the quest to provide an environment of well-being and minimize the impact of being in hospital, music appears to be a highly effective tool in the humanization process, helping to restore health. In fact, one of the reports during the observation of the visits in this study was of an improvement in a patient's oxygen saturation when his sister sang by his side during the visit. This relationship has not been properly documented, but we found a basis in a discussion about the role of music in hospitalized patients, which states that through mechanisms already known, it can be assured that musical sounds activate the brain's reward system, releasing neurotransmitters related to the sensation of pleasure, such as dopamine and serotonin, reducing pain, speeding up the recovery of patients, and therefore constituting an excellent resource for the promotion and recovery of health. This highlights the importance of this correlation in the evolution of patients who have attributes that help them improve, such as music and the arts as a whole.

Faced with this example of a humanization program and in view of its benefits and the hospital's needs, a similar initiative was set up at the Samuel Libânio Clinical Hospital in Pouso Alegre, Minas Gerais.

As with the "Remember me!" program, the motivation for setting up this program in this teaching hospital was not only the siblings' interest in getting to know the newborns, but also the psychological problems observed in the older children.

Parents reported feelings of guilt, abandonment, fear, anguish, sleep and eating disorders and difficulties with school and routine.

The reports of the newborns' families are decisive in expressing the importance of the project. The feedback was very positive, with a reduction in feelings of guilt, anxiety, abandonment, anguish and an improvement in school development and interpersonal relationships. In addition, the consolidation of a fraternal relationship and the establishment of a family bond were observed, as well as bringing the family closer to the hospital team.

Although some parents were initially a little wary of putting their older children and fragile newborns in contact, mainly because they were afraid that the first-born children would be more worried, the results were very positive. It was noticeable that, contrary to expectations, the children who were more aware of their sibling's situation came to understand their parents' greater absence better and began to take mature steps to help in any way they could.

In relation to health professionals, corroborating other studies, a limitation to the experience of humanization is a certain accommodation to the routine and wear and tear of ICU work. Taking into account the heavy and exhausting routine of the hospital environment, professionals in the area end up prioritizing the technical side and the efficiency of treatments to the detriment of the human side. It also turns out that the anxiety, anguish and suffering of parents "messes" with some professionals, who find it difficult to deal with painful situations when they are given bad news. For this reason, many of them clarify doubts and provide guidance only to the extent necessary, which has consequently reduced communication and the chances of exchanging knowledge and interacting effectively. Although they are aware of the importance of welcoming families, they find it difficult to put it into practice. In our study, this issue was significantly minimized by the effective work of the psychology department, which not only welcomed the siblings on visits and worked with the parents, but also approached the health professionals present, reinforcing their importance as carers of the hospitalized NB and, moreover, as collaborators in the care of the patient's entire family nucleus. In a study carried out in a neonatal and paediatric ICU in Maringâ, PR, all the professionals were unanimous in stating that the presence of parents with their child in the ICU is a decisive factor in optimizing the child's rapid recovery, and this is a positive point for them to mature in the idea of sharing with this new element (the parents) the space that was previously theirs alone, in order to guarantee the patient's effective recovery.

Thus, good care for hospitalized children requires guidance and the full involvement of the family in this process. Adopting intensive care aimed at stabilizing the child's hemodynamics, without dehumanizing care or disregarding the importance of the family for the child's recovery, is an attitude that should be taken by professional caregivers working in these units.

In this sense, we also saw the advantage of carrying out the study in the NICU environment of a teaching hospital, a place that by definition serves as a teaching and research field for students and professionals in medicine, nursing, psychology, physiotherapy and other health areas, who complement each other in caring for the patient. This experience of welcoming patients, even during the academic period, nurtures the formation of professionals with an outlook influenced by the humanized experience, who would be prepared to take this trend to the services where they may be hired and received as future professionals.

Given this panorama, it is clear that this project fits in perfectly with the attempt to humanize hospitals. Welcoming the siblings of newborns admitted to an Intensive Care Unit promotes a view of the patient that transcends the disease and manages to reach the entire psychological dimension that surrounds the hospitalized newborn and his or her family. Its importance and value are therefore evident.

7- Conclusion:

The experience of visiting small siblings in the NICU made it possible to ease the mother's anxieties and anxieties about her small child at home, dispelling feelings of guilt and abandonment of her healthy children. In addition, the young child feels like an active participant in their sibling's hospitalization process. The program for welcoming siblings of patients admitted to the NICU at Samuel Libanio Clinical Hospital was extremely important in reducing family stress, anxiety, feelings of guilt and anguish on the part of the older siblings, as well as keeping the family better informed about the health of the hospitalized NB and being able to adapt their routine to this situation. All of these benefits are an important reason to ensure that this program is g ven due credibility and continues to work.

The results categorically point to the importance of welcoming families as a relevant care technology for NICU practice. In order for this to happen, there is also a need to humanize working relationships within the Intensive Care Unit, with a view to welcoming families and including them as an element to be cared for. On the other hand, the study carried out at the teaching hospital proved to be important in training new professionals to focus their attention on humanization, to train in this area and to contribute to the extension of this project to other services in which they work.

In addition, we have come to raise debates and suggestions for greater support for the grandparents of hospitalized patients, based on the essential parental role that the figure of the "grandfather/grandmother" has taken on in the molds of the family and in the care of children, in order to include them in the care of this hospitalized newborn. We therefore hope that this study will serve as an impetus for projects that place the care of hospitalized patients' families as a driving force for action and results.

8- Annex 1 - Photos of visits by the siblings of patients in the Neonatal Care Unit of a Teaching Hospital

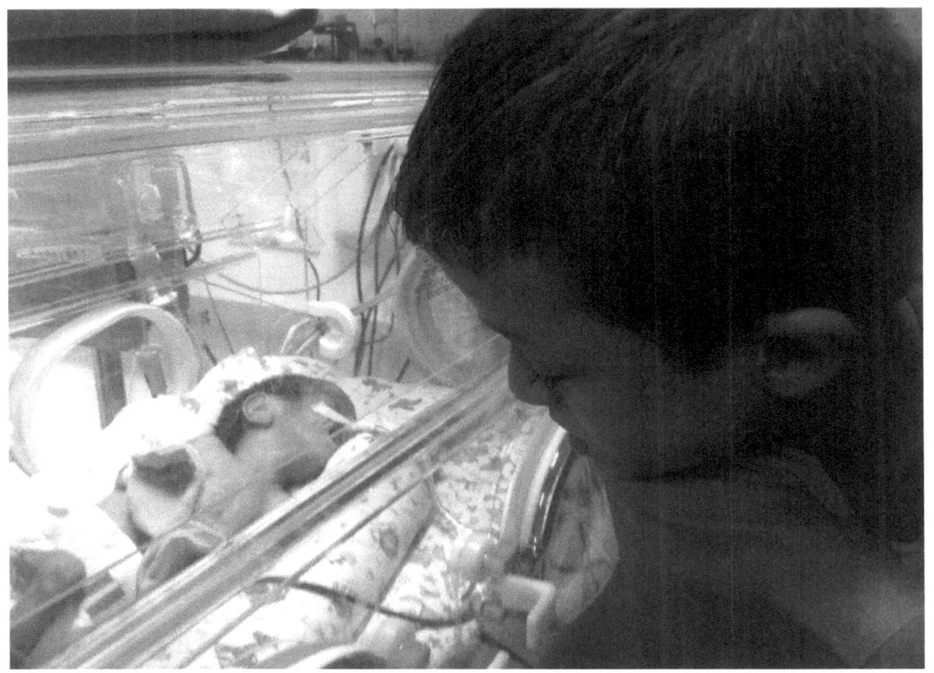

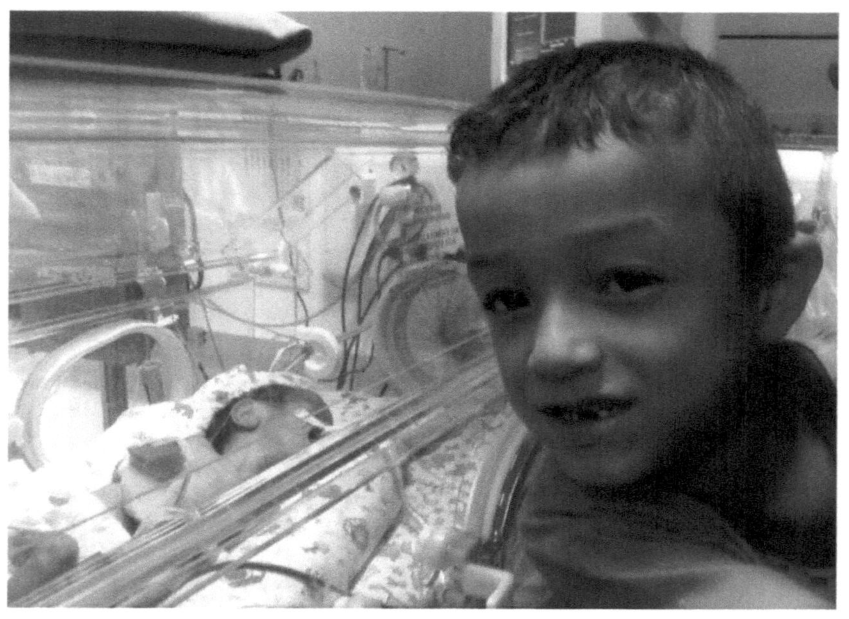

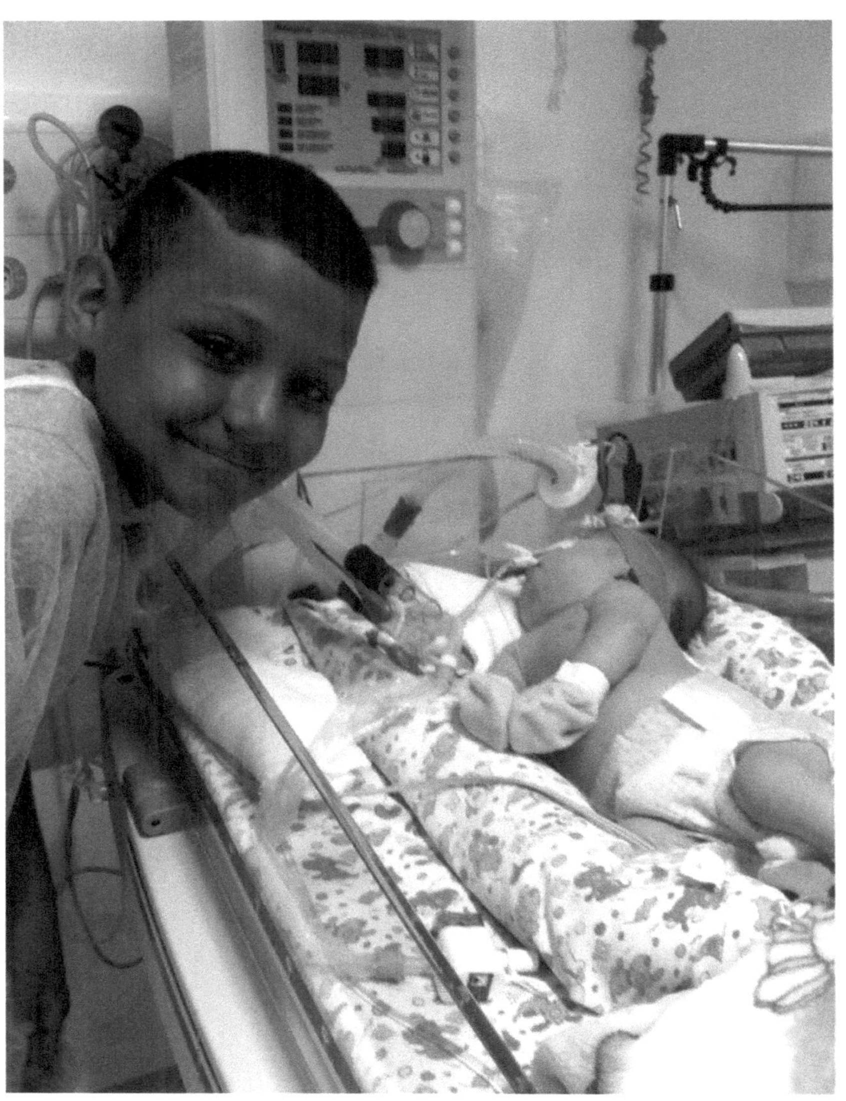

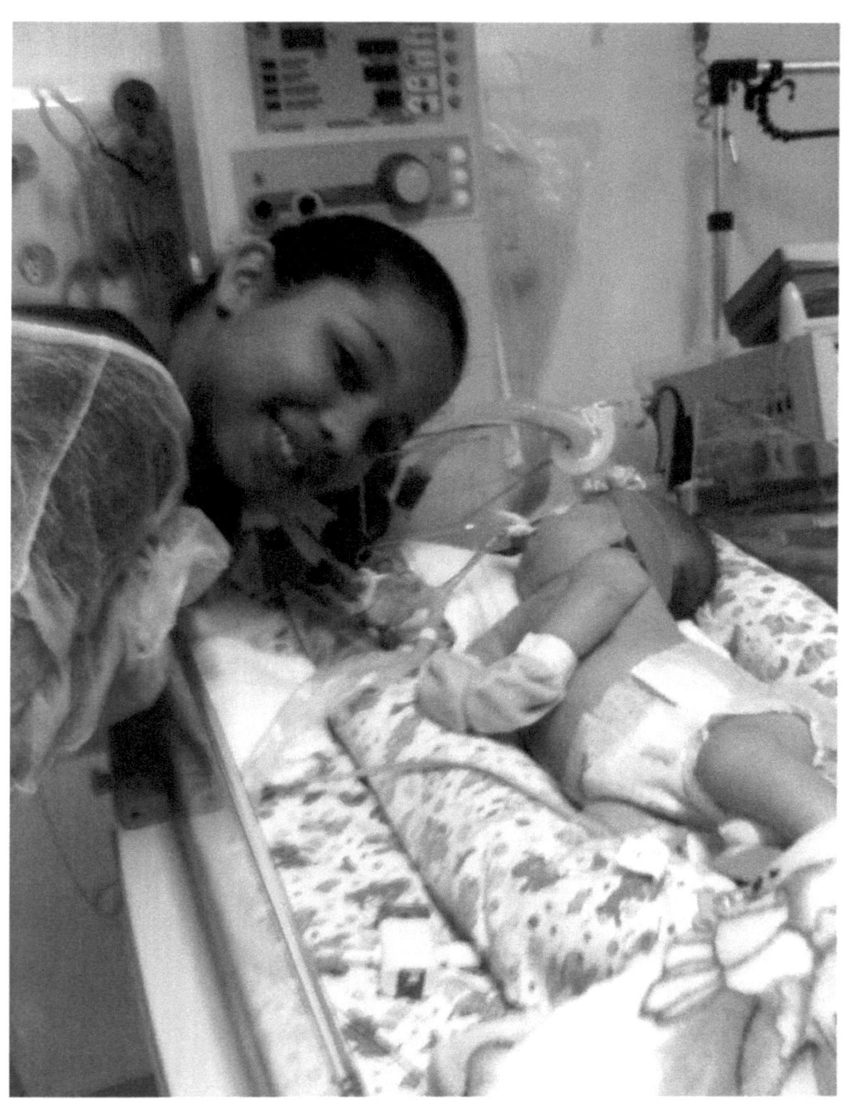

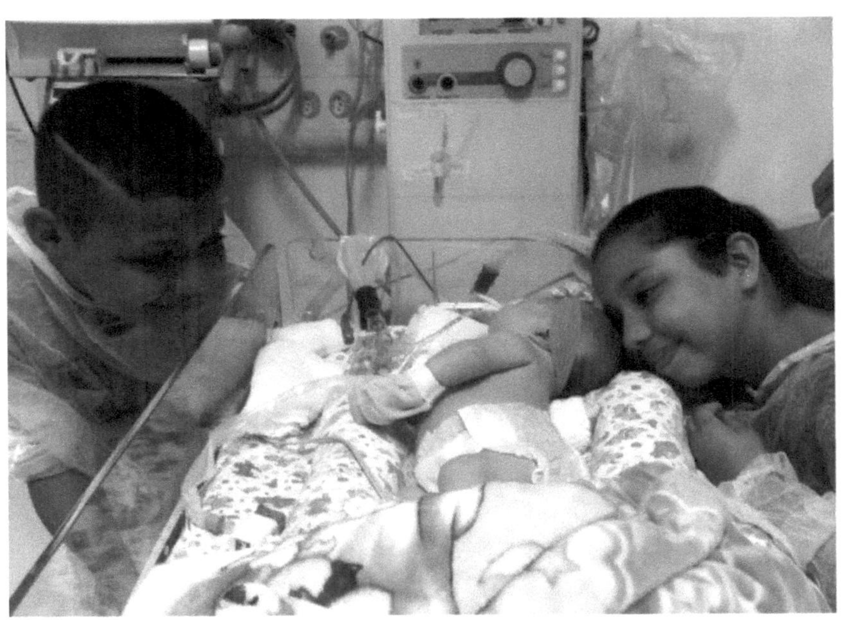

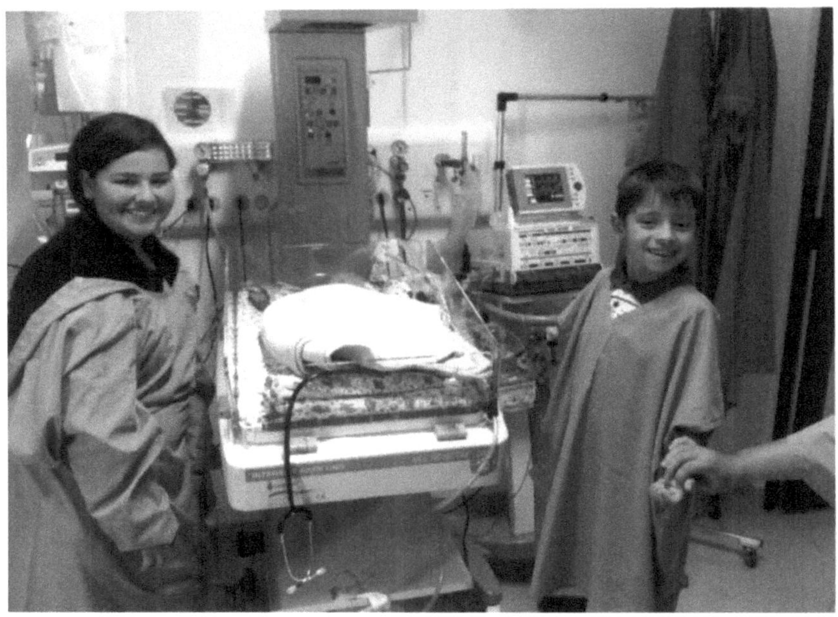

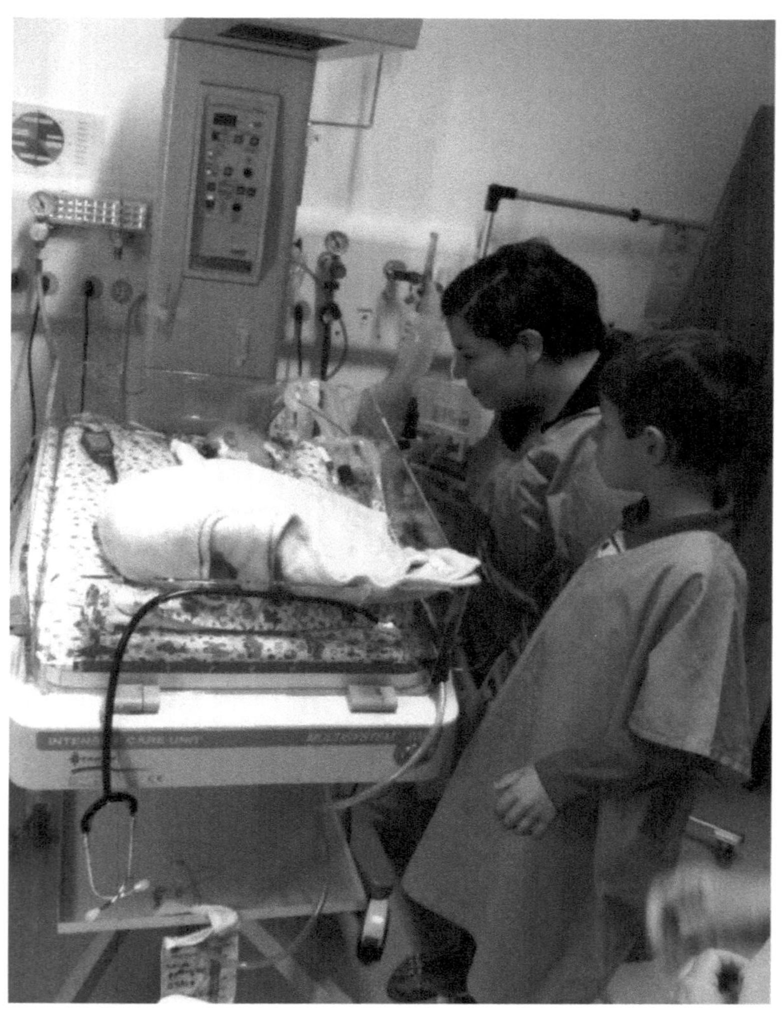

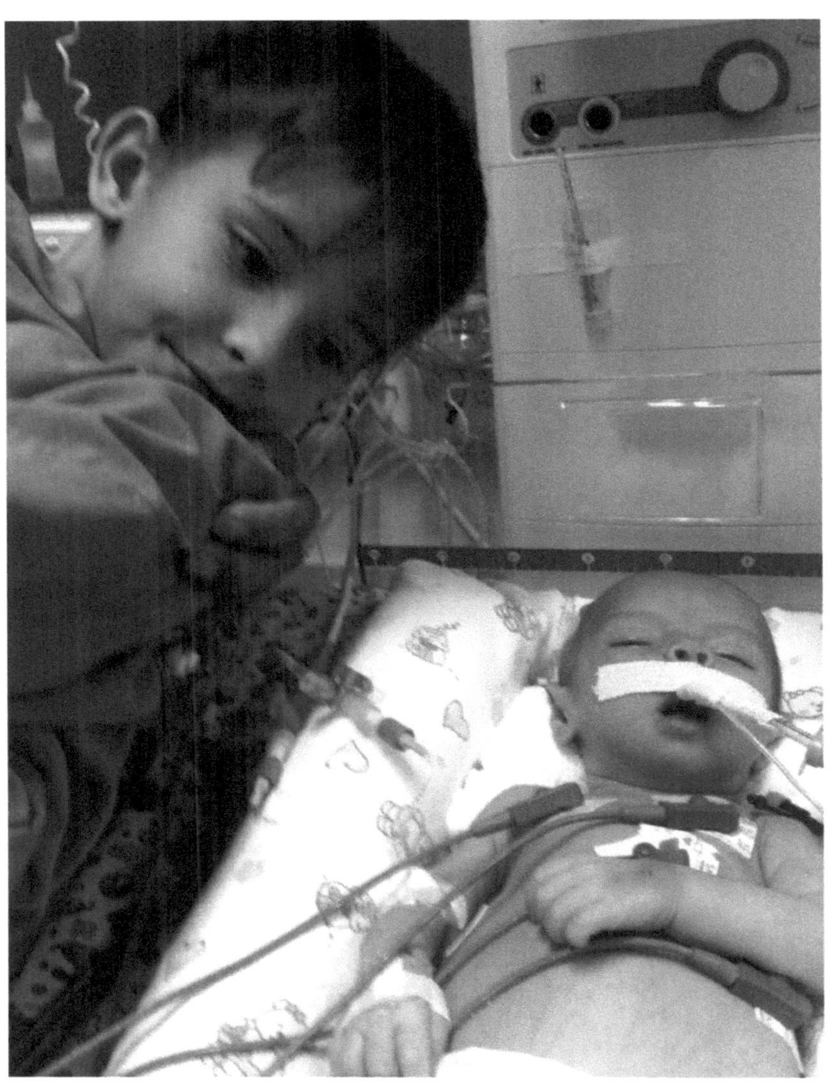

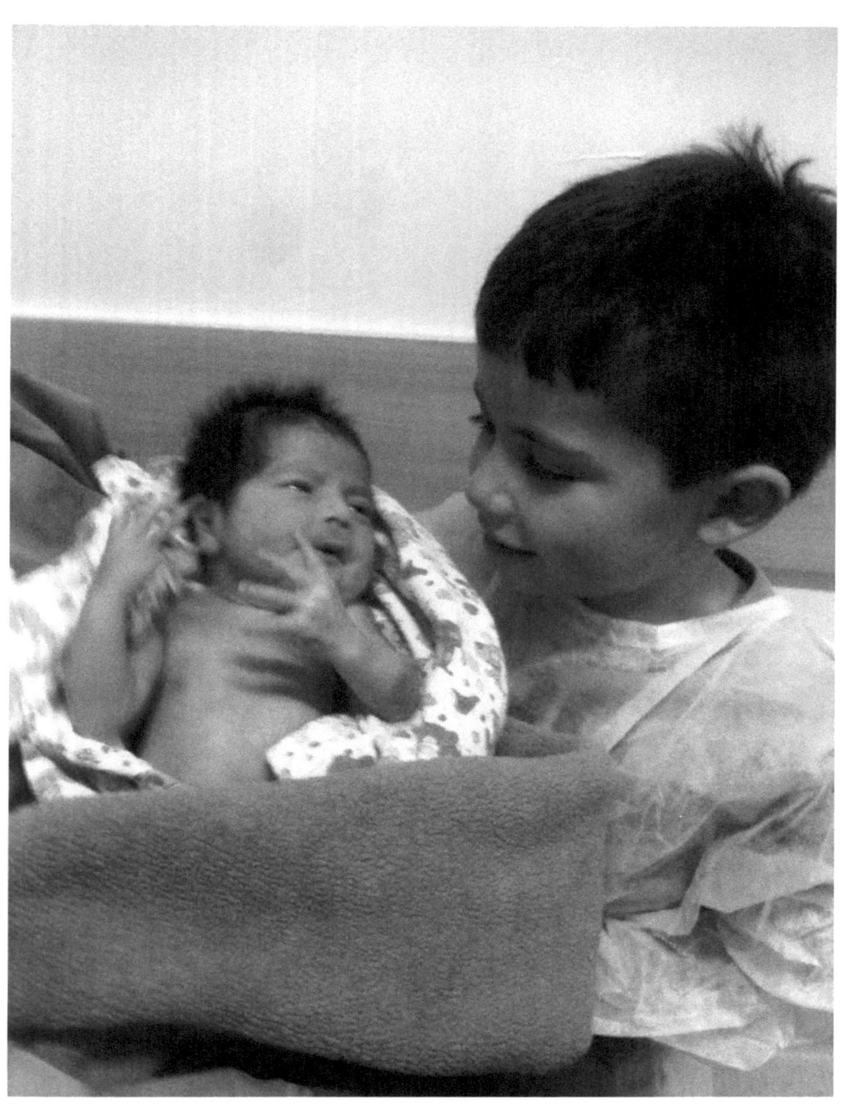

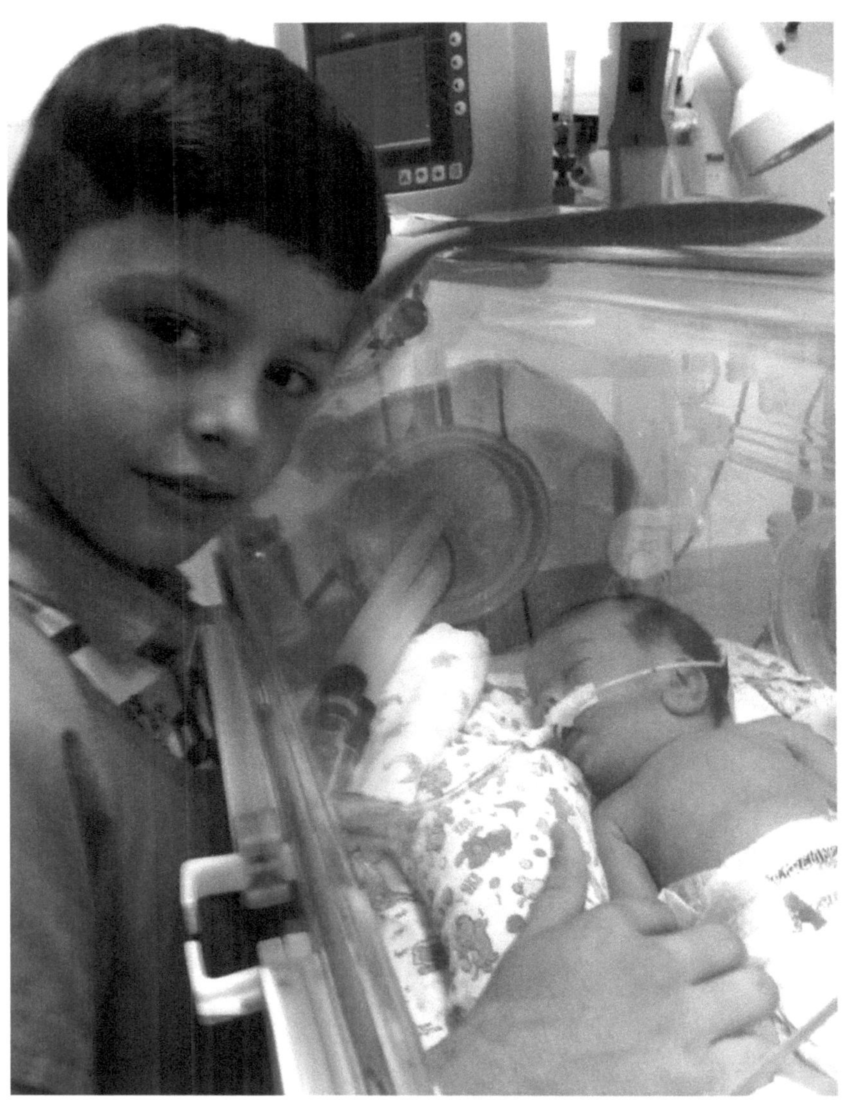

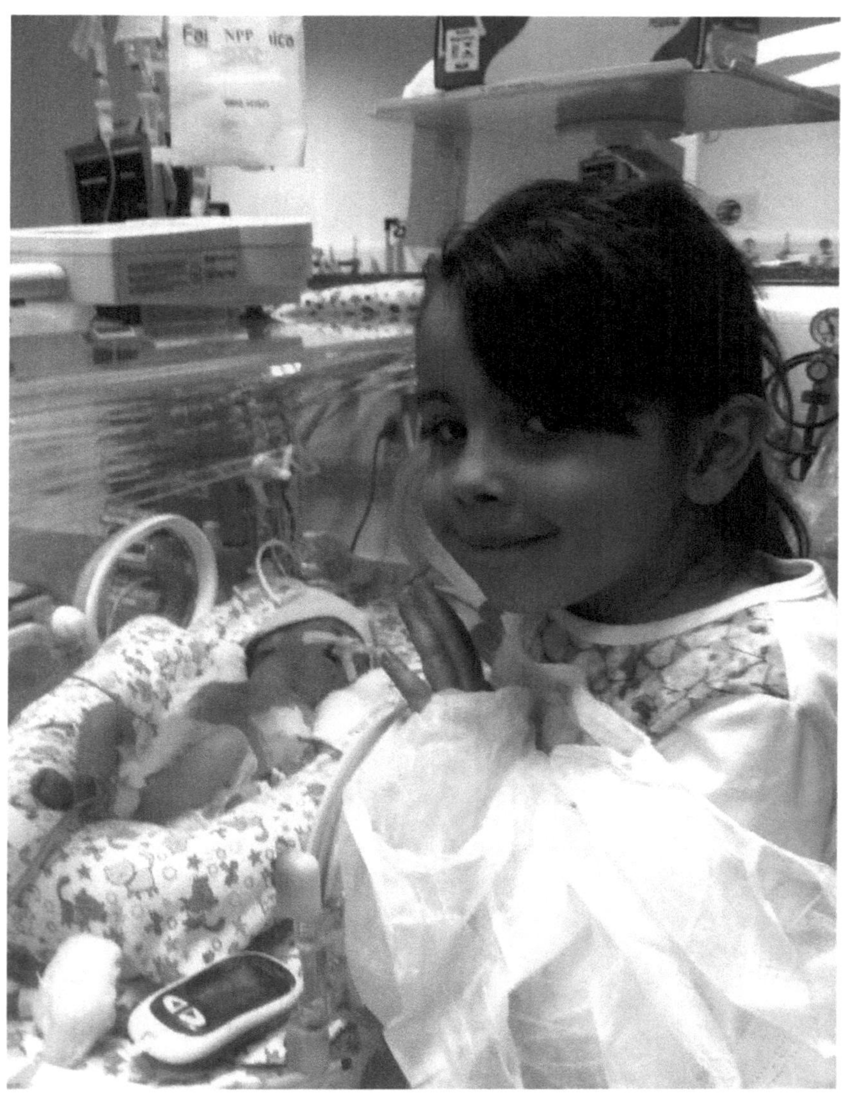

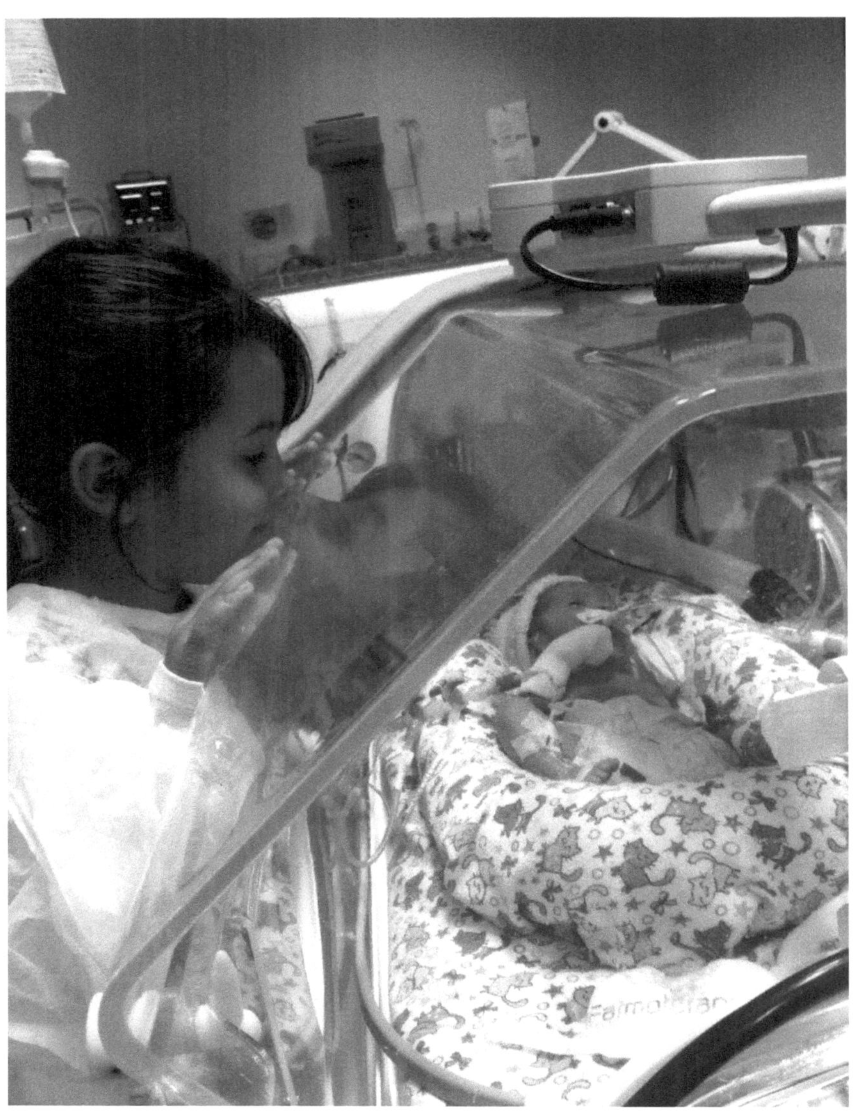

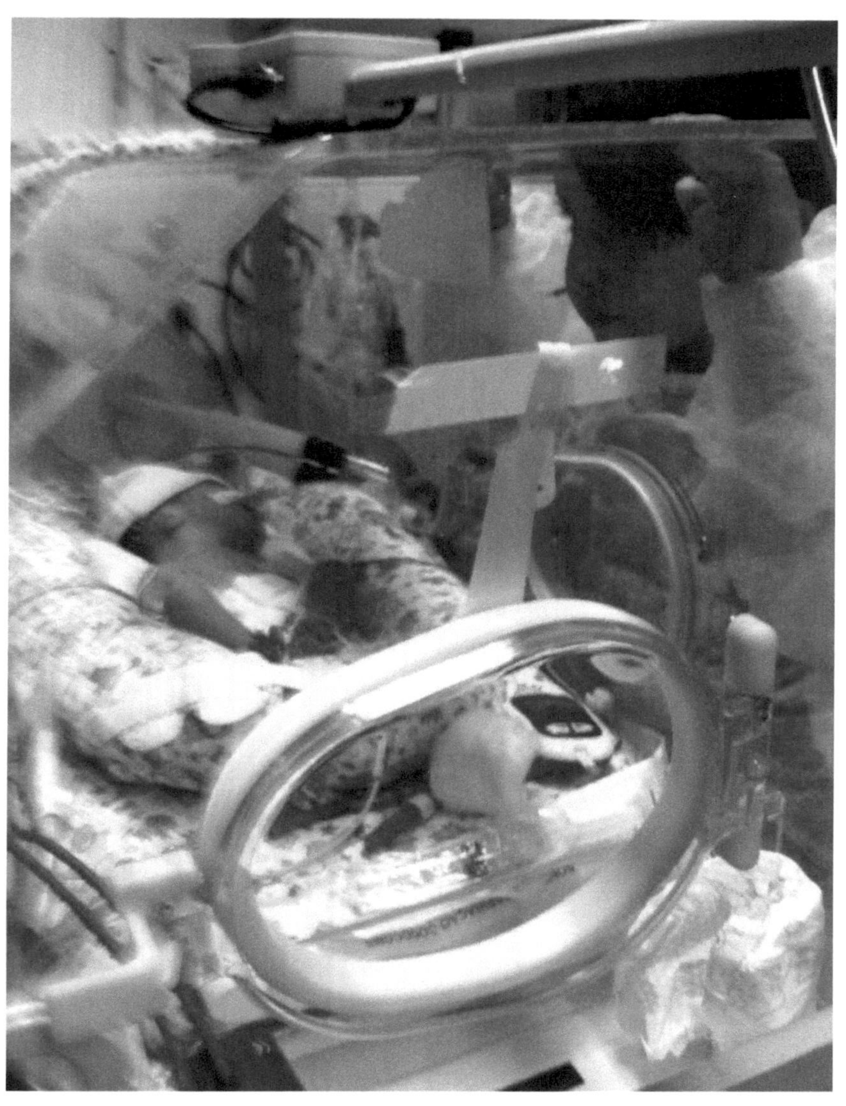

9- Annex 2 - Photos of visits by the siblings of patients in the Pediatric Intensive Care Unit of a Teaching Hospital

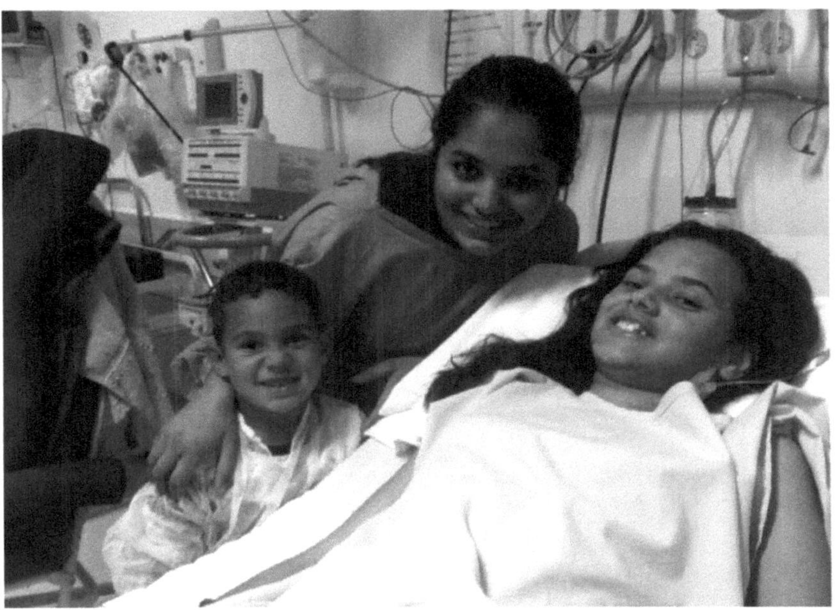

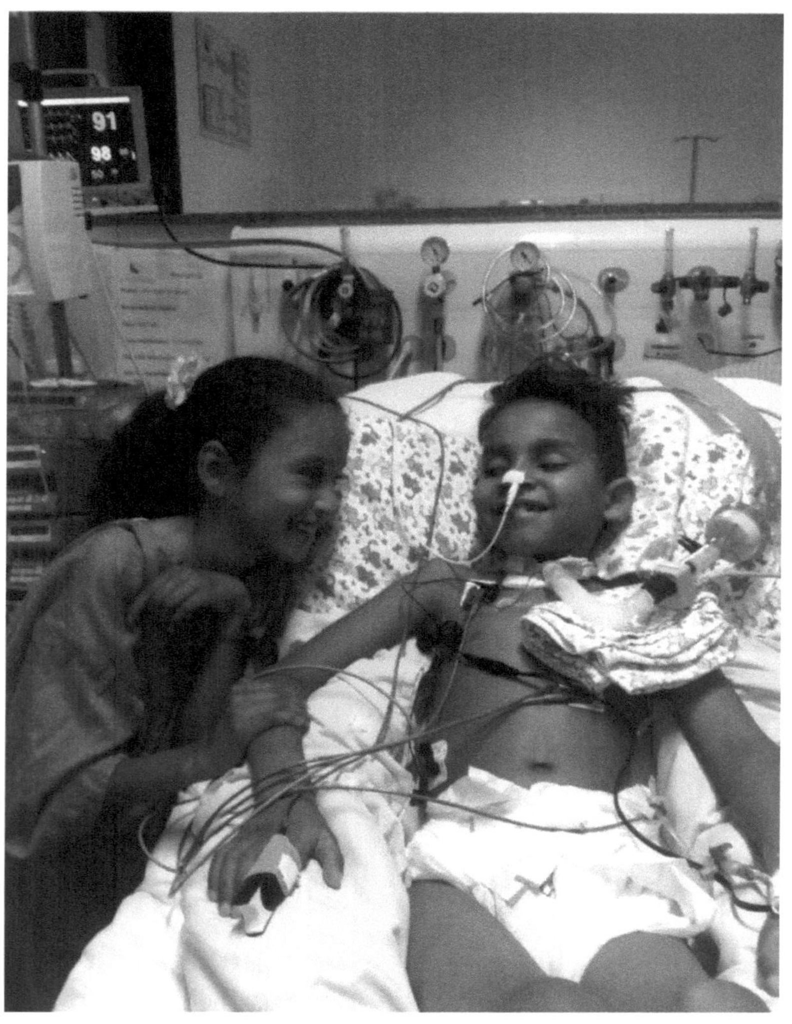

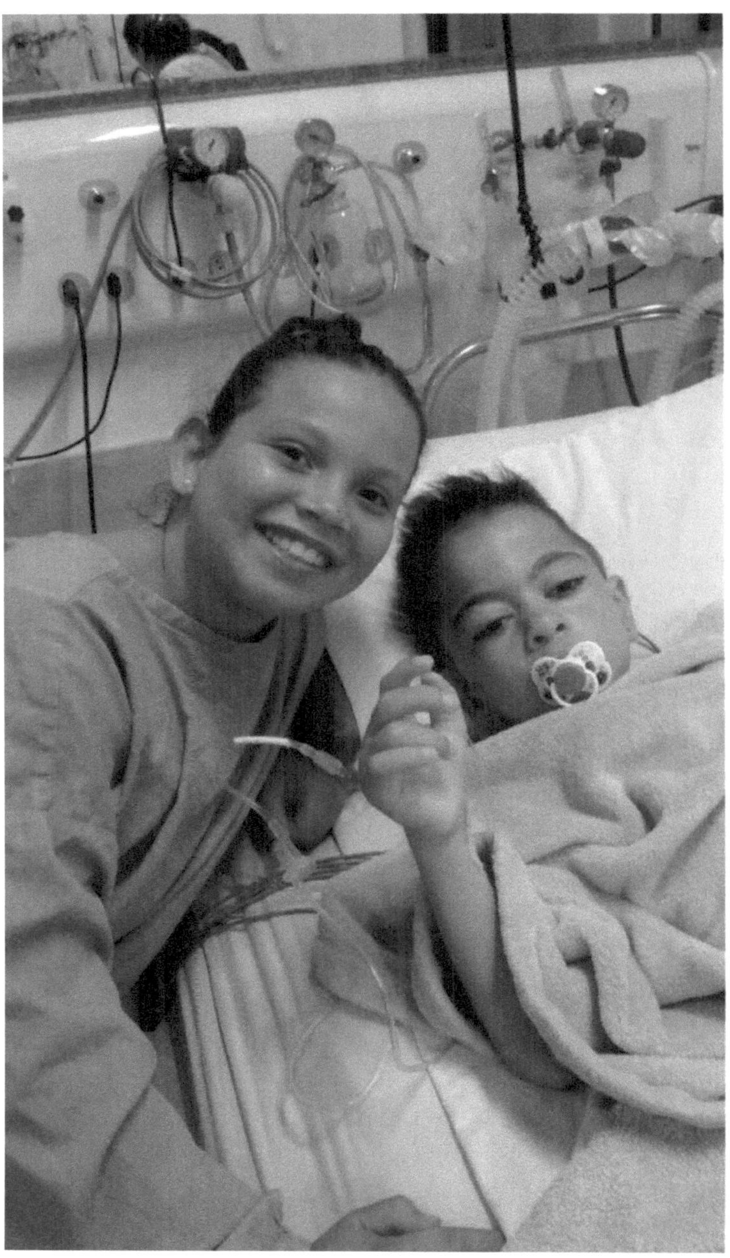

10- Bibliographical references:

BALTAZAR, Danielle Vargas Silva; GOMES, Rafaela Ferreira de Souza; CARDOSO, Talita Beja Dias. The **role of the psychologist in a neonatal unit: building routines and protocols for a humanized practice.** Sbph, Rio de Janeiro, v. 13, n. 1, jun. 2010.

GAiVA, Maria Aparecida Munhoz; SCOCHI, Carmen Gracinda Silvan. **Family participation in the care of premature infants in the neonatal ICU.** Revista Brasileira de Enfermagem, [s.i.], v. 4, n. 58, p.444-448, jul. 2005.

SOUZA, Adriany Miorini Vieira de; PEGORARO, Renata Fabiana. **The psychologist in the neonatal ICU: an integrative literature review. Saúde e Transformaçâo Social,** Florianópolis, v. 8, n. 1, p.117-128, 2017.

LEÀO, Livia Caetano da Silva et al. **"But aren't you going to bring your little sisters? Why did you win and leave them there?": siblings' experience of the premature birth of their baby.** Available at:

<https://www.lume.ufrgs.br/bitstream/handle/10183/104933/000939603.pdf?sequence=1>. Acesso em: 28 mar. 2018.

MOUSQUER, Paula Nunes et al. **Mâe, cadé o bebé? Repercussions of the premature birth of a sibling.** Available at:

<http://dx.doi.org/10.1590/0103-166X2014000400007>. Acesso em: 28 mar. 2018.

GARCIA, Daiana Fernandez. **Visits by siblings of newborns in the Neonatal Unit of a University Hospital in Porto Alegre, Rio Grande do Sul.** Available at:

<http://repositorio.jesuita.org.br/bitstream/handle/UNISINOS/6689/Daiana Fernandez Garcia_.pdf?sequence=1&isAllowed=y>. Acesso em: 28 mar. 2018.

ROCHA, Maria Cristina Pauli da et al. **Humanized care in neonatal intensive care: nurses' actions and limitations.** Saùde em Revista, Piracicaba, v. 15, n. 40, p.67-84, abr. 2015.

MEDEIROS, Juliana de Paula. **Mother-baby bond: possible encounters in a neonatal ICU.** Available at:

<https://repositorio.ufu.br/handle/123456789/17108>. Acesso em: 28 mar. 2018.

CAPARELLI, Estela; AMORIM, Alexandre. **Study warns about the situation of prematurity in Brazil.** Available at:

<https://www.unicef.org/brazil/pt/media_25849.html>. Acesso em: 28 mar. 2018.

PEREIRA, Alessandra Barbosa; FERREIRA NETO, Joao Leite. **Implementation process of the national humanization policy in a public hospital.** Trabalho, Educaçao e Saùde, Rio de Janeiro, v. 13, n. 1, jan. 2015.

MORSCH, Denise Streit; DELAMONICA, Juliana. **Analysis of the repercussions of the Program to Welcome the Siblings of Babies Admitted to the Neonatal ICU: "They Remembered Me!".** Ciência e Saùde Coletiva, [s.i.], v. 10, n. 3, p.677-687, 2005.

BACKES, Dirce Stein; LUNARDI, Valéria Lerch; LUNARDI FILHO, Wilson D.

Hospital humanization as an expression of ethics. Revista Latino-americana de Enfermagem, [s.i.], v. 14, n. 1, p.132-135, jan. 2006.

MOTA, Roberta Araùjo; MARTINS, Cileide Guedes de Melo; VÉRAS, Renata Meira. The **role of health professionals in the hospital humanization policy.** Psicologia em Estudo,, Maringà, v. 11, n. 2, p.323-330, maio 2006.

DESLANDES, Suely F. **Analysis of the official discourse on the humanization of hospital care**. Ciência e Saùde Coletiva, [s.i.], v. 9, n. 1, p.7-14, 2004.

LEPARGNEUR, Hubert. **Seeking a foundation for hospital humanization.** Mundo Saùde, [s.i.], v. 27, n. 2, p.219-230, abr. 2003.

Ministry of Health. **Kangaroo method.** Available at:

<http://portalms.saude.gov.br/saude-para-voce/saude-da-crianca/pre-natal-e-parto/metodo-canguru>. Acesso em: 14 abr. 2018.

SANTOS, Andréa dos et al. **Atençâo Humanizada ao Recèm-Nborn de Baixo Peso Mètodo Tanguru Manual Técnico.** Available at:

<http://bvsms.saude.gov.br/bvs/publicacoes/metodo_canguru_manual_t ecnico_2ed.pdf>. Acesso em: 10 abr. 2018.

MARTINS, Josiane de Jesus; NASCIMENTO, Eliane Regina Pereria do; GEREMIAS, Clàudia Koch; SCHNEIDER, Dulcineia Ghizoni; SCHWEITZER; NETO, Hilario Mattioli. **Welcoming the family in the intensive care unit: knowledge of a multi-professional team.** Rev Eletr EnFerm 2008; 10(4):1091-101.

LAMEGO, Denyse T. C.; DESLANDES, Suely F.; MOREIRA, Maria Elisabeth L..

Challenges for the humanization of care in a neonatal surgical intensive care unit. Ciênc. saùde **coletiva**, Rio de Janeiro , v. 10, n. 3, p. 669-675, Sept. 2005 . Available from

from <http://www.scielo.br/scielo.php?script=sci_arttext&pid=S1413-81232005000300023&lng=en&nrm=iso>. Access on 03 June 2018.

NASCIMENTO, Camila Aparecida Alves; CREPALDE, Neylson Joao Batista Filho. **Music as a resource in hospital humanization processes.** Formaçao Docente, Belo Horizonte, v. 7, n. 1, p. 24-35, jan./jun. 2015. Available at:<

http://www3.izabelahendrix.edu.br/ojs/index.php/fdc/article/view/756/pdf> Acesso em: 03 jun. 2018.

MOLINA, Rosemeire Cristina Moretto et al. **Family presence in pediatric and neonatal intensive care units: multidisciplinary team view.** Esc. Anna Nery, Rio de Janeiro , v. 11, n. 3, p. 437444, Sept. 2007. Available from

<http://www.scielo.br/scielo.php?script=sci_arttext&pid=S1414-81452007000300007&lng=en&nrm=iso>. Access on 03 June 2018.

MOLINA, Rosemeire Cristina Moretto; MARCON, Sonia Silva. **Benefits of the mother's permanent participation in the care of her hospitalized child.** Rev. esc. enferm. USP, Sao Paulo , v. 43, n. 4, p. 856864, Dec. 2009. Available from

<http://www.scielo.br/scielo.php?script=sci_arttext&pid=S0080-62342009000400017&lng=en&nrm=iso>. access on 03 June 2018.